Optimal Health

CHRIS M WILSON

Copyright © 2020 Chris M Wilson

All rights reserved. Your Optimal Lifestyle.

ISBN: 9798678321305

DEDICATION

This book is dedicated to my family. My mom and dad for pushing me to always give my best at everything I do. To my wonderful partner Vanessa for believing in me and supporting me no matter what happens.

OPTIMAL HEALTH

CONTENTS

	Introduction	1
	Why Your Health Matters	4
1	Picking the Right Type of Exercise for You	9
2	Creating a Healthy Environment	13
3	Setting Your Health Goals	16
4	Create a Schedule	20
5	Drink More Water	25
6	Improve Your Nutrition	29
7	Rest & Sleep	34
8	Track Your Progress	38
9	Mindset	42
	Outro	45

OPTIMAL HEALTH

INTRODUCTION

Thank you for reading this book. My goal is to help as many people as I can to create a healthy lifestyle through fitness and good nutrition. I am happy you are making a step in the right direction toward living a healthier life. Why should you listen to what I have to say? I have played competitive sports since I was 4 years old. Started lifting weights in gym class at age 14 and have been dedicated to exercising ever since. I have weight trained for over 15 years consistently, which led me to compete in fitness competitions for 4 years. This consisted of dieting for months on end along with training over 15 times a week. I continue to live a life dedicated to health and fitness to this day.

I want to warn you beforehand there are no shortcuts or secrets to creating a healthy lifestyle. This is a guide of practical information that I have experienced and tested over time. I have good days and bad days just like everyone else but understand that ***following a plan consistently is the key to reaching your fitness and life goals***. I know what it takes to make sacrifices to acquire something I want and commit myself to that cause. I have succeeded by learning from my failures and pushing myself every day to be better. It is my hope that you will enjoy and follow my 9-steps to creating a healthy lifestyle.

I am going to start off with a true story about a gentleman I know; we will call him Tom. Tom is a person who hasn't taken care of his body or health for a long time now. He's 70 years old is overweight, an ex-smoker, has diabetes, and Chronic Obstructive Pulmonary Disease (COPD). Symptoms include shortness of breath and coughing. He has been talking to me about a vacation to Antigua that he has always wanted to go on with his wife. The trip which he described in detail from the hot temperatures, sunshine, and the sound of the ocean crashing on the beautiful white sand beaches.

He rarely gets excited about much but when he starts talking about this once in a lifetime vacation, he becomes animated and enthusiastic. After saving for a long time to go on this trip he finally booked the tickets for him and his wife. He was so excited and couldn't wait to get there. He would finally enjoy the rest and relaxation he so deserved. Tom's trip was 7 days at a stunning resort on the island. He flew away and I wished him the best and said I wanted to hear all about his adventures upon his return. The next time I saw him I asked him to tell me all about it. "Was it the trip of a lifetime?" Tom didn't seem to have that same enthusiasm as before when he was describing his trip. He said quietly and barely looking me in the eyes, "I couldn't leave my room the entire 7 days. I couldn't breathe. I kept coughing and coughing. It was too humid, and my body couldn't handle the difference in the climate. I didn't get to experience anything at the resort and was miserable the entire time. My wife was out and about exploring and trying new things, but I was unable to even leave our room. I saved for that trip for a long time and wasn't even able to experience it." The reason I began with this true story is to remind every one of you, of the importance of your health. Without good health you may be cutting your life short as well as hindering your ability to enjoy the things that truly matter to you. By living a healthier lifestyle, you can make the most of your opportunity on this planet to live life however you choose to.

WHY YOUR HEALTH MATTERS

I would like to start with an important question - why does your health even matter? ***Health is defined as – the state of being free from injury or illness.*** Now this may be an obvious question to some but also harder to answer for others. Let's talk about why health matters to me and why It should matter to you as well. Rather than just sticking with the typical benefits of living a healthier life to look better and be more confident, let's dig a little deeper. With better health you will be able to experience great things throughout your life, look after those you care about, enjoy special moments with family and friends, or even travel and explore other parts of your country or even the world. You will be able to attend to what you value and seek most in life.

It may not seem important to you now if you are, for the most part, healthy. Many of us take our health for granted until we eventually lose it and it's too late to get it back. I want you to be proactive and realize that ***your health is one of the most important aspects of your life.*** It appears when we are younger, we work on ourselves more often through physical activity. Whether it is to get in better shape or improve our bodies for a given sport. As we get older our priorities seem to shift and work or family may seem to be an excuse to let ourselves give up and take the easy route.

Living a healthy lifestyle will enhance the areas you want to focus on in life and it will provide you with a sense of clarity. Whether it is your job, family, sports, or being able to live a life filled with energy and fun, being healthy is the key to doing all these things over the course of your entire life. Maybe you tell yourself you are too busy to dedicate an hour a day or a few hours a week to put towards your health. Or maybe you want to do more physical activities you enjoy but are lacking the time or knowledge to create a plan.

Currently we are living at a faster pace than ever before. We pile on "important tasks" day after day that are not all that important in the big picture. We make excuses to ourselves as well as everyone else about the obstacles in our way. Imagine your life 20 years from today without taking the time to look after yourself, what you eat, and how you take care of your body through physical exercise. Really imagine it, take some time now close your eyes and visualize what life would be like. I'm guessing it wouldn't look too great for you or others around you. Saying we don't have time to exercise and look after our bodies is like saying we don't have time to stop for gas in our cars. We will eventually be on the side of the road stranded and unable to get anywhere else. It just doesn't make sense in any aspect.

You get one life, one body, one opportunity to be at your best and live a life where you can be healthy, active, and fit. This does not mean you have to strive for an Olympic Gold medal or be the best in your field. I want you to improve your health so you can tackle whatever you want in life and be able to do it at the best of your own ability.

I have always been a big advocate of exercising through weight training and other activities, where I get a good sweat and raise my heart rate. It makes me feel clear, strong, healthy, confident, more energized along with reducing stress. Fitness helps me to recover from injuries as well as day to day activities quicker. Exercising just 3 times a week for a total of 3 hours has an endless amount of benefits to you and those around you. I understand going to the gym and weightlifting isn't for everyone and that's okay. We will go into more details in Step 1 about the different types of exercise you can do and what can work best for you in your current lifestyle. Here are 10 benefits that exercising and living a healthy life can do for you:

- *Increase chance of living longer*
- *Improved mental health and mood*
- *Boost brainpower*
- *Improve skin health*
- *Stronger bones, muscles, and joints*
- *Increase self-confidence*
- *Controls healthy weight*
- *Boosts energy*
- *Better sleep quality*
- *Strengthens cardiovascular health*

The list can go on and on about the benefits of exercise and living a healthy lifestyle. It's literally one of the best things you can do in your life that will give you incredible returns in the way of happiness, energy, and clarity. Exercise will also release **endorphins; these reduce your perception of pain as well as trigger a positive feeling in the brain.** The greatest benefit of all is not only does it improve your body and mind, but it allows you to excel in all the other vital areas in your life. Whether it's your job, hobby, or playing with your kids. You must prioritize and create a sense of urgency around your health and fitness. Our lives can change in an instant. By being healthy we can be better prepared to take on these changes in a positive way.

It doesn't take long until your bad habits are habits you have continued for 10 years without knowing it and now you will need to make some serious changes just to get back on a good path down the road. Our health is one of the most important aspects of our lives and without it we are unable to do the things we want to do and help others along the way. So please understand that you must prioritize your health in your life. Follow these 9 practical and actionable steps in this book. Before you know it, you will be well on your way to becoming the healthiest, happiest, and most energized version of yourself. ***Once you finish a section ensure you follow the action steps before moving onto the next section.*** There is space to fill in your answers following each step. You can also access printable documents online at www.youroptimallifestyle.com. The application of this book will create a strong foundation to empower you to succeed in creating a healthier life. Take the necessary time now to follow these steps to enhance your life!

"To keep the body in good health is a duty… Otherwise we shall not be able to keep the mind strong and clear."
-Buddha

STEP 1 - PICKING THE RIGHT TYPE OF EXERCISE FOR YOU

Our lives are unique and so are we which leads us into Step 1 - Picking the right type of exercise for you. When I was a child, I was fortunate enough to be involved in team sports. This was a great way for me to learn, grow, and stay active early on. I took part in all sorts of different sports such as baseball, hockey, basketball, volleyball, soccer, and lacrosse. In high school I was involved in a weight room class. I began learning about the human body and lifting weights in the gym. I loved the idea of changing my own body and the positive feeling it gave me during and after a session. I got hooked and started going to the gym 5 days a week to improve upon my previous week's weights. This has been my main form of exercise for the past 15 years – going to the gym following a set workout routine. This later lead me into the field of competing in Men's Physique. Pushing my body and mind to the absolute limit to be the best I could be physically and mentally. Now I include different types of exercise and activities into my life. Such as hiking, hot yoga, and snowboarding. Going to the gym and weightlifting is still at the backbone of it all.

Pro Tip - The tasks I do to get and stay fit are exercises and activities I enjoy doing.

This should be the root of your fitness programs as well – doing activities that you enjoy. You may be saying you don't know what you enjoy. You are going to have to be open minded to trying some new activities in your life. Some ways to find out what you may like doing are to; join a gym, go to your local community centre and see if they offer group classes, go on YouTube to lookup things that spark your interest, join a biking group, lookup Facebook groups with a fitness focus, or join a running club. There are lots of different ways to get good physical exercise. If you think you may want to play a sport you could try joining a league. If all of this sounds overwhelming to you try talking to friends or family to find out what they are doing to stay in shape.

This book is about helping you achieve fitness and health through ways that work with your life. We all have different jobs, schedules, incomes, and lives which affect when and where we have our free time. **Ideally you want to find ways to exercise which are fun and challenging.** There are many ways to get exercise such as: weightlifting, cardiovascular activities such as walking, running, biking, sprinting, or going on an elliptical. Sports such as volleyball, hockey, soccer, baseball, football, basketball, and lacrosse. Hobbies such as snowboarding, surfing, roller blading, skateboarding, and hiking. Group classes such as pilates, zumba, spin, yoga, hot yoga, core work, and strength/conditioning. There is a type of exercise for everyone out there.

Whether you are looking to push yourself hard and sweat or just raise your heart rate. Choose various ways to get exercise to keep things different and interesting for you and your body. If you include something like weight training and yoga, they will compliment each other well. As weight training will promote muscle growth and yoga will help speed up recovery and prevent injuries. I realize that walking on a treadmill for 30 minutes at the gym is not for everyone. Go outside and walk for 30 minutes instead, rain or shine and get the added benefit of being in nature.

Picking 2-3 different types of exercise and activities to incorporate into your life is great. I wouldn't recommend trying to pursue any more than that. If you try and do too much you will get overwhelmed and likely not achieve much. Everyone's life is different, and people will be at different stages in their fitness lives. The key here is to stick to exercises and activities in which you enjoy doing and are practical to fit into your current lifestyle. It's time to get out there figure out what you enjoy and make it a staple into your healthy lifestyle.

Action Step #1 – Pick 2-3 types of exercise you enjoy and write them down.
These will be the foundation of what you do for exercise. If you are just starting out it's time to try new activities and figure out what you like.

1._____
2._____
3._____

"It's not so much what we have in this life that matters. It's what we do with what we have."
-Fred Rogers

STEP 2 – CREATING A HEALTHY ENVIRONMENT

    Everything is easier when you have a supportive person or group behind you on your journey. This is important when it comes to fitness and health. Creating a healthy environment around you will help you to stay motivated and on track. ***I've been in the best shape of my life when training with a friend as an accountability partner.*** We motivate each other and it adds a competitive aspect to training. Having an accountability partner will help you both stay more consistent.

A good option is to find someone who also wants to create a positive life built on fitness and health. When you go to the gym, yoga class or play sports you schedule it in with your friend. This holds both of you accountable to each other. It also makes you both more likely to stick to a plan and follow through with it, without making excuses. Now an accountability partner can come in many shapes and forms. It doesn't necessarily have to be one person. You can hire a personal trainer who would hold you accountable for all your sessions. You can go to group classes each week, meet people in the class and start going with them. You can even attract these people to you from going to the places where you exercise already.

Pro Tip - A community or group can be invaluable in the support it can provide you along the way.

This is how I have created a health-oriented environment myself, by meeting people at the gym. Everyone there is focused on self-improvement and creating a healthier life. Some of the closest and longest relationships I have are people whom I met at the gym who have similar interests to me. A lot of us want to do everything on our own and couldn't be bothered with creating relationships along the way.

This leads us into our next key point that when you have your accountability partner/group and are seeing great results, *you start to change your environment and the community around you.* Your friends, colleagues, and people you associate with can affect what you do with your own life. This will make your journey much more memorable and exciting along the way. We want a long-term focus. Having some sort of accountability partner whether a friend, personal trainer, coach, or group class will help you stay on track for the long run to reach your best self. Surrounding yourself with a positive fitness and health environment will change the way you live your life daily.

Action Step #2 – Write down 1-2 people/class/personal trainer/coach/groups who could make a great accountability partner. This person or group will help be a supporting structure to your fitness community. If you are yet to have a good supporting group start building one around yourself.

1._____
2._____

"Never let the fear of striking out keep you from playing the game."
-Babe Ruth

STEP 3 – SETTING YOUR HEALTH GOALS

When starting anything in your life you need to set concrete tangible goals. These help you stay on track as well as give you something to aim for and achieve. With fitness and exercise there are many ways and targets in which we can set our goals. These could include goals such as nutrition, weight loss, muscle building, physical goals, frequency of training or more specific like to see your six pack. Without goals we are wandering aimlessly. This can lead us to coast more which will give you minimal results.

Pro Tip - One of the most powerful tools when setting your goals is to write them down on paper.

We are more motivated and driven to accomplish something when we set the specifics and a deadline. This not only gives you something visual to see everyday and keep you on track but it's another way to hold yourself accountable and create clarity of what you want to achieve in your fitness life. I recommend setting no more then 3 health goals at a time. This will keep you focused on what's truly important to you. Making it more likely that you will achieve them in a timely manner. **Setting fewer goals will allow you to have a more focused vision to reach them.**

Now you may be asking, what's the best way to set goals? There are many ways and different forms to goal setting with endless books on it. If you have a system that already works for you then great, you can stick with that. I personally like to follow the **SMARTER** goal setting system devised by Michael Hyatt. It's an acronym that stands for:

Specific
Measurable
Actionable
Risky
Time-keyed
Exciting
Relevant

One example of a goal following this system would be:
- **Lose 5 lbs in 8 weeks (by this date)**

Specific – Lose 5 lbs
Measurable – 5 lbs in 8 weeks
Actionable – Go to gym 4 x week for 8 weeks starting this week
Risky – Aggressive goal must lose over ½ lb per week
Time-keyed – An 8-week time frame to reach goal, write down the end date
Exciting – I've wanted to weigh under 200 lbs for over 5 years now
Relevant – Losing this weight will ensure I feel healthier about myself

Some more examples of great health goals:
- **Gain 3lbs of muscle mass in 8 weeks**
- **Go to the gym 4 x week on set days**
- **Go hiking twice per week**
- **Play hockey 3 x week in a league**
- **Bring healthy food to work 5 x week**

Your goals can be whatever you want them to be regarding your fitness life but be sure to follow the **SMARTER** system for best results. *Goal setting will help you stay motivated, have a clearer vision of what you are striving for, and allow you to track your progress.* Sometimes we may not reach our goals on time or perhaps never if we set our sights too high and that's okay its part of the journey. If you fail to reach a deadline or are struggling to achieve a certain goal, go back to the drawing board, see what can be done differently and adjust that goal moving forward. Goal setting is critical to achieve what we want to in our fitness lives. Whether you are young or old having goals written down will improve the likelihood of achieving what you want sooner.

Action step # 3 – Write down 3 health goals.

That you would like to achieve in the next 1-6 months following the **SMARTER** goal setting system. Keep these nearby and refer to them daily before you exercise to keep you on track.

1._____
2._____
3._____

"It is better to take many small steps in the right direction then to make a great leap forward only to stumble backward."
— Proverb.

STEP 4 – CREATE A SCHEDULE

After you have completed the first 3 steps – # 1 picking the right type of exercise for you, # 2 create a healthy environment and # 3 have set your 3 health goals you are ready for step # 4, which is to create a schedule for your exercise. Many people think that to live a healthier life, they can buy a gym pass and go when they are free. Hoping it will all fall into place after that. Unfortunately, this is usually not how it works from my experience. People are motivated towards the goals they have set and are excited at the beginning which gives them a burst of enthusiasm. This excitement and energy allow them to be consistent for the first month or so. Then as time goes on, they begin to fall back into the original bad habits they had developed before they decided to make a change for the better.

Creating a schedule that fits with your lifestyle will help you to stay on track. ***If you want to accomplish your goals, get into great shape, and feel amazing you must schedule your fitness into your life like your job is scheduled.*** We must look at making health and fitness part of our lives everyday. Not just a quick fix to lose some weight and rebound back over time. It is more important than the outside physical looks most people often tend to focus on, especially the younger generations.

This leads us to scheduling in a plan for your type(s) of exercise and activities. Think of your job, most of the people these days working a normal day job work Monday to Friday between the hours of 8:00 a.m. to 5:00 p.m. You know when to leave your house in the morning to drive or take transit to work. You know when your breaks are and lunchtime. Lastly you know when to call it quits and leave to go back home that evening. (I do understand that some people's jobs vary times and places day to day like my own). But for a good amount of people there is a routine in place each week around that schedule. You have a schedule, a plan, something to stick to, whether you feel like going to work or not your hours are set. You are expected to show up and do your job at the given times. This is how I want you to treat your health and fitness with a set schedule built with structure.

Pro Tip - It works best to stay on track and stay consistent when we stick to a set schedule week after week, month after month.

A set schedule and routine has allowed me to train all these years with extreme consistency. Plans can change sometimes, and you may have to miss your workout to deal with an emergency. This is part of life and how it goes sometimes. You want to take your own health seriously and stick to your schedule at all costs. ***A schedule for your fitness will hold yourself accountable each day and be a priority near the top of your list of to do's.***

As I stated earlier that without your own health it can be tough to focus or help others throughout your life. Now you may be wondering how much time a week you should be dedicating to your types of exercise. This will differ for everyone and their goals/lifestyle. I like to get a minimum of 5 hours of exercise or physical activity each week. That's about 5 x week 1 hour per session whether it's at the gym or in a yoga class. Some weeks I will be more active than 5 hours if I incorporate a sport like snowboarding a couple of times that week. My weekly activity level could be well over 10 hours then.

A typical week for me might look like:

Sunday – Rest
Monday – Weight training 10:00 a.m. – 11:00 a.m.

Tuesday – Hot Yoga 9:30 a.m. – 10:30 a.m.
Wednesday – Snowboarding 9:00 a.m. – 12:00 p.m.
Thursday – Rest
Friday – Weight training 10:00 a.m. – 11:00 a.m.
Saturday – Weight training 1:00 p.m. – 2:30 p.m.

It will look different for everyone, but the point is you want to create something that will work for you in your life. ***I would recommend getting at least 3 hours of exercise per week minimum.*** This should be realistic for most people to achieve. Maybe the best time for you to get exercise is at 6:00 a.m. at home with resistance bands before work. Or it could be 7:30 p.m. after dinner when you have some free time. Not only do you want to schedule in the days but also write down the time and duration of the exercise. This keeps you from making up excuses and missing a session. Write them into your planner if you have one and/or into your phone calendar. ***You are scheduling a session for you to be a healthier version of yourself.*** Stick to it and make it a top priority for that given day. Creating a schedule for your exercise will keep you consistent and accountable. It's such an easy task and will have positive lasting affects on your health over a lifetime.

Action Step # 4 – Create your ideal fitness week.

Schedule in what exercise(s) or physical activities you want to do on given days, along with the start time and duration. Be sure to write it in your planner and/or into your phone's calendar.

Sunday
_____

Monday
_____

Tuesday
_____

Wednesday
_____

Thursday
_____

Friday
_____

Saturday
_____

"The only impossible journey is the one you never begin."
-Tony Robbins

STEP 5 – DRINK MORE WATER

One of the most overlooked aspects of achieving a healthy lifestyle and feeling great is drinking water and staying properly hydrated. Our bodies are made up of anywhere between 60% - 80% of water depending on where we are in our given lives. Without water we would not survive.

It is essential to life and we require it daily for proper body functions. **Hydration is one of the easiest steps to living a healthier life.** Although it is one of the most overlooked by those trying to make a positive change in their lives. Many people may feel symptoms of dehydration – when your body does not have as much water as it needs daily. Some of these symptoms include – thirst, hunger, dry mouth, headache, and muscle cramps. Water intake for individuals can vary quite a lot depending on age, sex, activity level, climate, etc. Everyone will need a different amount.

Pro Tip – Drink 500mL upon waking to hydrate your body immediately.

I would recommend for adult females to drink a minimum of 2L per day and adult males at least 3L per day. If you live a highly active lifestyle, are an athlete or someone who sweats a lot, anywhere from 4L plus per day may even be necessary. I tend to drink between 3-4L per day but when I was competing 5-6L per day was normal. Once you get into a good habit of drinking a set amount daily assess how you feel mentally and physically. Adjust your intake to where you feel your best daily. Some of the key benefits to staying properly hydrated are:

- Keep joints lubricated
- Deliver nutrients to cells
- Prevent infections
- Boost immune system
- Help organs function properly
- Maximize physical performance
- Help energy levels and brain function
- Help prevent headaches
- Aid in weight loss

While these are only some of the benefits there are many more. I like to have a filled 1-liter water bottle beside me wherever I go during any given day. This helps me ensure I drink enough water.

Get a 1-liter bottle that you like and fill it in the morning. Make it a goal to drink 2-4 bottles per day. This will keep you hydrated and acts as an easy way to track your intake. You want to set yourself up for success. *From my experience having a 1L bottle is the best way to keep your water intake high.* I personally enjoy drinking water. It tastes great, is refreshing and makes me feel energized and clear. A lot of people I know do not have the same love for water. They dislike the taste or think it's boring and couldn't be bothered to drink a cup or two a day. This is one bad habit you will have to change immediately if you want to be at your best health for years to come.

Beware of drinks that will dehydrate you such as pop, alcohol, or coffee. If you drink these make sure you are drinking an additional 2 cups of water for each cup you drink on top of your daily intake. *Some ways to help make water more appealing and tastier to drink are by adding lemon, lime, cucumber, mint, or orange slices to your bottle.* These foods can add great benefits to the water you are drinking; like adding valuable nutrients and minerals needed by your body, boost your immune system, and help with digestion. You will be creating a healthy, refreshing, and hydrating drink that is cost effective.

The bottom line is you must be drinking enough water for your body to operate at its best and desired levels. Start at the low end of what I have recommended and adjust as necessary, depending on how you are feeling. Staying properly hydrated will give you tons of benefits that you may have thought came from elsewhere. Our bodies are mostly made from water so do yourself a favour and stay hydrated everyday!

Action Step # 5 – Get a 1-liter reusable bottle.

Make it a daily goal to drink 2-4L of water each day depending on you and your activity level. Track your intake for a week. Assess how you feel each day and adjust the amount if necessary.

Sunday
_____

Monday
_____

Tuesday
_____

Wednesday
_____

Thursday
_____

Friday
_____

Saturday
_____

"Lighten up, just enjoy life, smile more, laugh more, and don't get so worked up about things."
-Kenneth Branagh

STEP 6 – IMPROVE YOUR NUTRITION

This is one of the most important pieces to living a healthy lifestyle – nutrition. One way I like to compare diet and exercise is the 70-30 rule. This means that to reach your fitness, health, weight loss, weight gain goals it will be based on 70% nutrition and 30% exercise. If you want to lose 5lbs in 8 weeks by solely going to the gym 5 x week, it will be more challenging on yourself and your body if you do not incorporate good nutrition.

Eating healthy food is the fuel your body needs to function at a peak level. When people think about eating healthy the first things that come to mind may be; diet, restriction, costly, time consuming, boring, and unappealing. This can be true for some people or some athletes depending on what their goals are. But for most we need a better understanding of the foods we should be eating to promote healthy living.

While I competed in fitness shows I would typically diet on a set plan between 12-16 weeks continuously. This was extremely calculated, every meal I ate was weighed to the gram. I did not have any options to eat anything else off the plan. This was what worked for me in that given time. Bodybuilding can have some of the most extreme nutrition restrictions than any other sport in the world. I did this to succeed in a specific sport but to live a healthier life we need to improve our daily nutrition decisions.

I do not want extreme restrictions for you nor do you have to have them to get in better shape and improve yourself. I was an athlete competing to push myself to the absolute limit through nutrition and training. For the average person it should look a lot different from this. It all depends on your goals and what you want to achieve. Everyone will have different foods they prefer or like best. The key is in building habits daily. ***Nutrition will be the main leverage you have regarding weight loss, weight gain, and being the healthiest version of yourself.***

I'm not going to go into huge amounts of detail in this book on nutrition. This is meant to be a practical guide to creating a healthy lifestyle not a diet or nutrition manual. But I will give you some tips and tricks on how to choose healthy foods and ways to stay on top of your nutritional goals. It all starts with the grocery store and buying the right foods for you. Nowadays you can order your food online right to your door. This can be a great way to eat healthy as it stops you from buying random unhealthy items you do not need while you shop.

Pro Tip - Avoid grocery shopping while you are hungry.

Many of you probably know how this feels already, you tend to buy a lot of unhealthy foods you want in that moment. It is easier to say no once at the grocery store to unhealthy foods than many times at your house when they are in the cupboard. If you do end up going to the grocery store shop around the outside perimeter of the store for most of your items. This is where you will find most of the whole foods like, vegetables, fruits, meat, eggs, etc. If you are getting it in a bag or box it's processed and likely contains a huge list of unknown or hard to pronounce ingredients.

Learn to take the time to read the nutrition labels of the foods you're buying. Compare two products side by side, maybe one has more sugar than the other. A great way to start eating healthy is to incorporate lots of colourful fruits and vegetables into your meals and snacks. Eating lean meat, fish, and some complex carbohydrates such as brown rice, oats, sweet potatoes, or yams will keep your protein and energy levels up. There is a lot of information online that points to quick diets and tricks to eating better. I have always found sticking to the basics by eating smaller portions of real whole foods work best. The food you eat daily should not make you feel restricted or unhappy. You want to make healthy nutrition habits a new way of your life. A general recommendation would be to stick to making food at home at least 5 days a week. Eating homemade healthy food throughout the week would be a fantastic start to improving your nutrition.

Something I have adopted other the years is meal prepping. This will not only help you save money from going out and eating but also ensure you are making smart healthy choices beforehand. Food preparation ensures your making smart decisions and are prepared for the coming days. You could meal prep all your food for your work week Sunday afternoon including your lunches and all your snacks. This also relieves a lot of pressure during the week as you have everything packed in your fridge ready to go for the upcoming week.

Another important item you will want to consider is portion sizes when eating. The average portion sizes at restaurants these days is usually a lot more then we should consume in one sitting. I would recommend having smaller meals throughout the day with snacks in between. When you have a meal, half of your plate should be veggies, one quarter lean meat and the other quarter is for complex carbohydrates. This is a good rule to follow for many people.

I suggest picking up a set or two of various sized Tupperware packs. This will help greatly in terms of creating healthy eating habits. You will have a place to put healthy meals and snacks on the go. Remember good nutrition is the key ingredient to creating a healthy lifestyle. It should not be overly restricting or boring. Your body is running off the fuel you put into it so make sure you take care of it to feel energized, happy, and healthy.

Action Step # 6 – Make up a grocery list of at least 15 healthy items.
Including all the food groups to get for this coming week. Use Tupperware packs to hold your meals/snacks in for the week. Start incorporating these foods into your daily eating habits.

"You must expect great things of yourself before you can do them."
-Michael Jordan

STEP 7 – REST & SLEEP

Proper rest is important for your body to repair itself. From my experience it is best to have a minimum of 2 rest days per week to function at an optimal level. These days should consist of little to no exercise or cardiovascular exertion. Rest is also crucial to living a healthy life and reaching your fitness goals. This is when your body repairs itself and builds back stronger than before. If you do not allow your body time for the necessary rest it needs, you will be limiting your overall progress. Your body will not operate at its highest level.

This brings us to one of the most important forms of rest we need to live our healthiest lives – sleep. Sleep is vital for everyone looking to live a healthy life. While sleep times can vary between everyone *a good general rule to follow is to get at least 7-8 solid hours of sleep per night.* You want to create a good routine for when you go to bed and when you wake up. For me I like to sleep at 11:00 p.m. and wake up at 7:00 a.m. 8 total hours. I can function on less but usually require 8 hours if I want to feel my best and be clear everyday. To get a good night sleep every night make sure your room is cool and dark. Limit caffeine intake and avoid big meals or a lot of fluids a few hours before bed.

Pro Tip – Turn off all your screens such as your phone and T.V. at least 30 minutes before you sleep.

Some of the benefits of sleep include keeping your heart healthy, reduce stress, reduce inflammation, increase energy and alertness, improves memory, and helps the body repair itself. With proper rest and sleep you will be able to live your healthiest life. It is important from professional athletes to anyone who wants to be clear minded and energized daily. Find the right number of hours for you and your life. You should wake up feeling reenergized.

It is a good idea to build a weekly routine around your sleep. Ideally you want to be going to sleep and waking up at the same times each day. On weekends this may differ. Try and follow a schedule for at least 5 days of the week. This creates a good pattern for your body. It will respond well when you need to sleep and when to wake up. Play around with your sleep routine/schedule to find what works best for you.

For most people, their work schedule will likely dictate at least when they wake up in the morning. If you work at 8:00 a.m. during the week and wakeup at 6:30 a.m. then going to bed at 10:30 p.m. on weekdays would work well. Find a sleep schedule that you like, that works with your lifestyle and allows you to feel great upon waking up each day.

If you are not sleeping long enough each night you will be limiting your body's ability to function the next day. If you can rest a minimum of twice a week from your exercise routine and get 8 hours of sleep per night you will be well on your way to feeling your best.

Action Step # 7 – Create a sleep schedule for your ideal week and follow it for 2 weeks. Ex. Monday to Friday 10:00 p.m. – 6:00 a.m. Saturday and Sunday 11:00 p.m. – 8:00 a.m. Take a minimum of 2 full rest days from exercise per week – scheduled into your ideal fitness plan from Step # 4.

Sunday
_____

Monday
_____

Tuesday
_____

Wednesday
_____

Thursday
_____

Friday
_____

Saturday
_____

"You get in life what you have the courage to ask for."
-Oprah Winfrey

STEP 8 – TRACK YOUR PROGRESS

You have set your goals, have a strong exercise/sleep schedule implemented into your life, are hydrated, and eating well which has allowed you to feel great everyday. But how do you know how far you have come? This is where tracking your progress comes in. To help us see where we have come from and what we have accomplished.

I like to follow a weekly and monthly review plan. This is a self review to see what you did well and what you can improve on. Everyone's review may differ slightly as it depends on exactly where you are trying to go and what you are trying to achieve. There are many ways to track your progress as well. **Ways to track your progress include – weight, body fat calculation, and measurements.** Using different systems to track your progress is ideal. Sometimes your weight may not be decreasing although you are still achieving positive results like reducing your body measurements. This is a typical scenario when someone is building muscle. You can also calculate your BMI – Body Mass Index which takes into a person's age, height, weight, and sex.

Pro Tip – Get a blank notebook to keep all your fitness tracking information in. This can be referred to at anytime for quick reference.

Other ways to track your health along your journey is to take notes how you are feeling. You can do this mentally by thinking about how you feel before or after your exercise. Or you can record how you are feeling in a fitness journal or notebook. This is a fantastic way to get your results on paper. It can be a useful tool to allow you to understand when you're feeling good or have less energy than normal. Some people may not see the value in tracking their progress. Stating their goal is not to become an athlete it's to live a healthier life. **It is important to see where you have come from and all that you have accomplished along the way.** Sometimes it can be hard for us to see how far we have come. The changes seem to come slowly making it hard for us to notice.

It is extremely useful to see where you could improve from the previous week or month. Maybe you missed 2 workouts last week because you were too tired after work. If you track this, you can figure out ideas or ways to improve and make next week better. Maybe you can workout earlier before work on those 2 days next week before you are too tired to go. Without weekly/monthly reviews it can be difficult to know what we have done well and what we have not. Tracking your progress is helpful for average fitness enthusiasts and competitive athletes alike.

When I was working with a fitness coach, he would hold me accountable for my actions and review my progress. Tracking your progress along your journey is important. Pick a couple of ways that are accessible to you like weighing in each week and taking measurements every 2nd week. Make sure you are taking the time to step back and review the good and the bad. **We must learn from our previous mistakes and improve week by week.** This will lead you to a healthy life where you feel happy and excited. When we can see how far we have come it makes us feel great to keep going and pushing further.

Action Step # 8 – Focus on 2-3 areas of measurement such as weight, body measurements, and bodyfat.
Record your weight once per week and the others every second week. Get a notebook or journal to record your weekly/monthly fitness review in.

Week 1
_____

Week 2
_____

Week 3
_____

Week 4
_____

Week 5
_____

Week 6
_____

Week 7
_____

Week 8
_____

"Every second you have on this planet is very precious and it's your responsibility that you're happy."
-Naval Ravikant

STEP 9 - MINDSET

The most important step when it comes to creating a healthy life and achieving anything in life starts and ends with your mindset. ***Mindset is defined as the established set of attitudes held by someone.*** My mindset has always played a significant role in my accomplishments. I have always been good at sports and other activities I enjoy doing but never the best. When I competed, my edge was not my genetics it was my mindset. This allowed me to go all the way to bring something special to the stage. I can focus extremely well on a task and do what is necessary over a long period of time to get positive results.

You must stay 100% committed by staying positive and believing in yourself throughout the entire journey. Whether you want to stay focused for an hour at the gym or on your sport for years, you must be mentally prepared to do the task at hand and do it to the best of your ability. You must have a clear and positive outlook and be able to visualize yourself having already achieved your goals. This will help you in times of resistance to keep pushing forward. If you want to be proud of your body and confident you must feel like that now. If you want to be a champion act like one.

Pro Tip - You have what you want already, the power of your mind. The trick is to focus on what you want and believe you can get there.

Let your mind guide you to where you want to go. I want you to have a positive and optimistic view. We must train our mind like we train our bodies. Empower yourself and your mind through meditation. This step is so important in fitness and in life. Most people are looking for some magic pill or secret to help them along the way. Unfortunately, there isn't such a thing. Your mental attitude will help you to achieve anything you want in life. You must first create your healthy life within you. Act with intention like someone who is healthy and create positive habits. Use your mind to change your world for the better. Use your mind to make healthy choices to live a happier, healthier, and more abundant life. Use your mind to help you achieve - Optimal Health.

Action Step # 9 – Believe in yourself and what you can accomplish.
Write down 3 positive affirmations regarding yourself and your life. Don't wait to be the person you want to be - Act and feel as that person now.

1._____
2._____
3._____

"It always seems impossible until it's done."
-Nelson Mandela

OUTRO

If you made it this far you are well on your way to creating a healthy life. This is something you must live. Something that is a part of you. It is about making the right decisions every day to promote living your best life. It will not be easy. It will not be quick. But if you commit to creating a healthy life by following the 9 steps, it will pay off with more dividends than ever imagined.

Chris Wilson

"Whether you think you can, or you think you can't – you're right."
-Henry Ford

www.youroptimallifestyle.com

Printed in Great Britain
by Amazon